Ketogenic

MW01595440

ACKNOWLEDGMENT

I express my profound gratitude to my wife Amanda, whose contributions and support toward the success of this book cannot be quantified.

She has been very supportive and understanding, I am so grateful for that.

TABLE OF CONTENTS

Chicken skewers with rosemary buttermilk.

Low carb stuffed zucchini and BBQ chicken.

Hot dog with BBQ bacon cheese

Avocado salsa diet with grilled salmon.

Skewers of shrimp scampi

Northern fried chicken recipe.

Onion soup with London broil

Burgers stuffed with caramelized onion and Brie.

Yogurt sauce with chicken souvlaki

Shrimp of pesto.

The Barbeque ribs jerk.

Low carb cheese roll ups and salami.

Jalapeno poppers

Low carb Mediterranean eggs recipe.

Low carb perfect guacamole

Barbeque shrimp wrapped with keto-bacon

Hot dog keto-recipe

Low carb pups and dogs recipes.

Potato salad low carb recipe

Low carb keto corn bread

Low carb cauliflower salad and shrimp

Pine nuts and feta with grilled zucchini.

Flow carb cobb salad

Broccoli salad

Balsamic reduction with salad of tomato mozzarella.

Pecan vinaigrette (toasted and grilled asparagus)

Smith apple slaw.

1. Chocolate Barbeque sauce.

2. Mango Barbeque sauce with smoky tomato.

3. Vinaigrette herb with garlic.

4. Pesto of green radish

5. Barbeque sugar-free sauce.

6. Recipe of pesto

7. Gorgonzola butter with ribeye steak

8. 30 seconds Caesar dressing

Lemon bar dessert

Chapter one

INTRODUCTION

First and foremost, congratulations for taking this bold step to move forward in this process of gaining a healthy and positive weight loss. Indeed, I'm happy that this ultimate guide book will be of immense help to you, for your family, friends, colleagues and relatives.

Thanks a million for having a copy of this amazing recipe keto-book that was designed to help you with many ketogenic recipes, grills, desserts, BBQ's, Keto-drinks and juices which can be used at home, events, picnics, parties, celebrations and other festivals that demand low carb, high fat delicious diets or drinks. I really got your back here!

I know of a lot of people that have tried all they could necessarily do to lose some pounds of flesh including purchasing both online and offline weight loss pills, practicing rigorous and stressful exercises, surfing the internet day and night for the latest weight-loss strategy among many others which may not contained in the context of this book. In all these practices, litter or no success is actualized. Rather, there seems to be an upsurge in weight even after following the prescribed weight loss regimen. Hope this sounds familiar?

Now how will you see it if I tell you that you can effectively lose those extra weights and enjoy a better and healthier life just by abiding FAITHFULLY on a change in diet and drinks that are in this guide which I have thoroughly researched over the years and found that they are effective and efficient in giving you the actual result and body stature you want: A perfect diet that you can use anytime and any day for your household and offshore events (perhaps in situations where you have guests that are restricted to ketogenic recipes). You can steal a glimpse from this book and wow them... lol!

Ketogenic diet is the only ideal recipe that can help you actualize this aim. It has main focus on a recipe that is high in dietary fat consumption, low carbohydrates and moderate protein content. This low carb diet enables you to have a healthy weight loss following intense burning of fats that occurs daily even while you are sleeping.

This book will emphasize more about the ketogenic diet and how it works. Most importantly, there are detailed list of new amazing recipes that you gonna learn their preparation: how to get started with preparation of Keto main dishes, side dishes, salads, snacks, dips, BBQ's, grills, desserts, appetizers diets and many more – *All in the Keto-style.* When you are done with these recipes well-prepared, you will see the positive changes that will surprise you.

Let's get started!

CHAPTER TWO

GETTING STARTED STEP BY STEP

These awesome Keto diets are fantastic and delicious to prepare as it comprises amazing recipes that are ideal for your Christmas/festive celebrations and picnics including parties alike and for your normal household dishes. Low carb desserts, condiments, side and main dishes, appetizers and even drink are all covered in this great book. Hence there is no hesitation inviting your friends over for a party and revealing to them these amazing lists of diets in the keto-way.

This list of keto-diets have been categorized which makes it easier for you and can also enable you with your diet planning. You can easily match or mix one or more keto recipe from any category and you will be good to go for any celebration or events pertaining your health most especially as regards your weight.

1. Keto BBQ and Main Dishes
2. Low carb snacks, Dip and Appetizer Diets

3. Low Carb Salad and Side Dish Recipes

4. Drinks recipes (Low Carb)

5. Picnic Low Carb Recipe.

CHAPTER THREE

KETO BBQ's AND MAIN DISH RECIPES

1. Chicken skewers with rosemary buttermilk.
2. Low carb stuffed zucchini and BBQ chicken.
3. Hot dog with BBQ bacon cheese
4. Avocado salsa diet with grilled salmon.
5. Skewers of shrimp scampi
6. Northern fried chicken recipe.
7. Onion soup with London broil

8. Burgers stuffed with caramelized onion and Brie.

9. Yogurt sauce with chicken souvlaki

10. Shrimp of pesto.

11. The Barbeque ribs jerk.

1. CHICKEN SKEWERS WITH ROSEMARY BUTTERMILK

OVERVIEW:

This is a very mouth-watering dish that has combined fresh rosemary buttermilk with a dressing mix of valley ranch all over. Its aroma is amazing buh oh boy you gotta watch out to see how your family will enjoy this diet to the fullest. This diet is wonderful all day long buh it is very good to eat as we approach Xmas or for our parties and picnics. The rice or green fresh salad is served with layers of chicken making it really yummy and enticing.

INGREDIENTS:

Chicken breast (boneless) (2kg)

Butter milk (One cup),

Virgin Olive oil (one-third cup)

Worcestershire sauce (Two tablespoon)

Valley ranch dressing (one Oz)

Fresh pepper (Half teaspoon)

Minced rosemary (Two sprigs)

PREPARATION:

1. Dissect your chicken into bits (one-inch cubes).

2. Gently arrange the chicken on skewers after soaking first for 30 minutes in water if you are using bamboo.

3. Put marinde onto the chicken and refrigerate for about 60 minutes.

4. Let your skewers be grilled for 20 minutes after pre-heating your grill to medium temperature.

5. Serve and enjoy your meal immediately.

B. LOW CARB STUFFED ZUCCHINI AND BBQ CHICKEN

OVERVIEW:

This dish is very easy to prepare most especially when you book your meat from Rotisserie chicken republic which is what I'm doing. Once it is baked after adding it to the zucchini, you will automatically get a good texture and flavor. Give it a trial this Xmas or any of your outings and give me a hint of what you think. One thing I like about this dish is that it is easier to reheat on your microwave.

INGREDIENTS:

Sugar ketchup (one-third cup)

Cider vinegar (one-quarter cup)

Onion powder (One teaspoon)

Yellow mustard (Two teaspoon)

Granulated sugar (Two tablespoon)

Liquid smoke (one-quarter teaspoon)

Mayonnaise (Two tablespoon)

Chopped cilantro (two tablespoon)

Chopped red onion (Two tablespoon)

Raw corn kernels (one-quarter cup)

Cooked chicken (Two cups)

Zucchini (Two)

Shredded Jack cheese (Half cup)

PREPARATIONS:

1. Whisk the cider vinegar, onion powder, mustard, sweetener, mayonnaise, liquid smoke and ketchup in small bowl. Put the

corn kernels, cilantro and red onion and then mix very well after adding the shredded chicken.

2. The zucchini should be dissected lengthwise with the centre portion scooped out and then season with pepper, salt. Heat for 5 minutes till it softens.

3. Fill up the zucchini with the same composition of BBQ chicken mixtures and bake it for half an hour at 360 degrees till the cheese melts after spraying the shredded cheese on it.

4. Serve and enjoy your meal.

This recipe has 4 servings and each serving contains 27g protein, 17g fat, 6.5g carbs and 290 calories.

C. HOT DOG WITH BBQ BACON CHEESE

OVERVIEW:

One of the most interesting and unique recipe is the hot dog with BBQ Bacon cheese which is super tasty, easy and an amazing way to prepare for prepare something delicious. Give this meal a trial in your subsequent Barbeque and I bet you, you will be happy you did.

INGREDIENTS:

Hot dogs (eight)

Gouda cheese (eight slices)

Bacon (sixteen slices)

BBQ sauce (Half cup)

Tasted hot dog buns (Eight)

PROCEDURE:

1. Slice the hot dog (each of them) lengthwise and fill with your cheese.

2. Use two slices of the pre-cooked bacon to wrap your hot dog and hold the bacon in a fixed position with your toothpicks. Decorate using your most favorite Barbeque sauce.

3. Grill gently the sides till your bacon becomes crisp, the cheese

becomes melty and the hot dog sweating.

4. Enjoy your amazing and unique diet

D. AVOCADO SALSA DIET WITH GRILLED SALMON

DESCRIPTION:

This is another delicious and healthy recipe with enormous flavors and aromas; it's very quick and simple to cook. This recipe is mouth-watering with incredible flavors which you must give a trial.

INGREDIENTS:

1. Salmon (two kilogram)

2. Olive oil (one tablespoon)

3. Salt (one teaspoon)

4. Ground cumin (One teaspoon)

5. Paprika powder (one teaspoon)

6. Chili powder (Half teaspoon)

7. Black pepper (one teaspoon)

8. Sliced avocado (one)

9. Sliced red onion (half)

10. Lime juice (half-cup)

11. Chopped cilantro (two tablespoon)

12. Salt.

PREPARATION:

1. Mix properly your paprika, onion, cumin, chili powder, salt and then rub your salmon fillet with the seasoning mix and olive oil.

2. Put in the refrigerator for a period of 45 minutes; mix your lime juice, cilantro, onion, avocado and salt in a medium bowl and cool.

3. The salmon should be grilled to your desired taste (I do mine for 5 minutes)

4. Sprinkle your meal with avocado salsa.

5. Serve and enjoy.

This serving contains 21g protein, 19g carbs, 22g fats and 366 calories.

E. SKEWERS OF SHRIMP SCAMPI

OVERVIEW:

I am really excited to bring this meal your way this period for you to cook at home. This is one of the tastiest and easiest sources of protein. I prepare this shrimp every festive season or any of our outings which makes my children to give it a tag "#Festive Shrimp#.

INGREDIENTS:

1. Large raw shrimp (One pound)
2. Lemons (3)
3. Kosher salt (Half teaspoon)
4. Black pepper (Half teaspoon)
5. Red pepper flakes(one-eight spoon)
6. Parsley butter with garlic: Butter (Three tablespoon), Minced garlic (Two cloves), Dry white wine (One

quarter cup), fresh parsley (One-quarter cup)

PREPARATIONS:

1. The butter should be melted by heating it in a medium heat microwave.

2. Put the white wine after adding your garlic and steam for a period of 3 minutes combining it with the molten butter.

3. For the skewers, slice your lemons and thread your shrimp onto your skewers and then spray with your red peppers, salt and black pepper evenly on the skewers.

4. Grill for 5 minutes till the shrimp becomes pink and then gently

brush the parsley butter all over your shrimp.

5. Serve and enjoy.

F. NORTHERN FRIED CHICKEN RECIPE

OVERVIEW:

This diet is great and equally amazing recipe which is enriched with a lot of nutrients and can be prepared easily. With about six servings, you gonna try this recipe and I bet you that you will enjoy it.

INGREDIENTS:

1. Chicken leg (5kg)

2. Salt (one teaspoon)

3. Garlic powder (one teaspoon)

4. Paprika (one teaspoon)

5. Coconut flour (one cup)

6. Oil.

PROCEDURE:

1. Mix the pepper, garlic powder, salt, chicken and paprika. Massage with your hands those spices inside the chicken to make it well-coated.

2. Refrigerate for a period of 60 minutes.

3. After seasoning of the chicken, ensure to toss it very well with the coconut flour which gives it a coat.

4. Fry the coated chicken in a large bottomed frying pan till it becomes crisp or becomes golden.

5. Check the meat temperature using a thermometer which should be about 165 degrees. Although you can ascertain this temperature by cutting the meat into pieces which ideally should not be pink prior to servings.

6. Serve and enjoy

G. ONION SOUP WITH LONDON BRIOL:

OVERVIEW:

This recipe is quite ideal for celebrations and it's a quickie because it can be cooked within 30 minutes. The timing could be adjusted based on your desired choice and temperature can be checked using a thermometer which should be around 150 degrees Fahrenheit.

INGREDIENTS:

London broils (one and half pounds)

Olive oil (2 tablespoon)

Onion soup seasoning (one-quarter cup)

Dried onion flakes (one-quarter cup)

Onion powder (one teaspoon)

Sea salt (half teaspoon)

Palm sugar (Half teaspoon)

PREPARATION:

1. Use the oil to rub your meat and then coat very well using your onion soup mix.

2. Using an aluminum foil lined by a baking sheet, broil the meat on each side till you get your desired taste or texture.

3. Remove from heat and allow settling for 7 minutes; slice thinly on top of the seasoning.

4. Enjoy!

H. BURGERS STUFFED WITH AND BRIE

OVERVIEW:

There is nothing so satisfying and enriching to a wonderfully-prepared juicy hamburger with amazing toppings. Honestly, this mixture of caramelized onions and brie is a perfect match. When I told my wife about the idea, she could not help salivating over the whole stuff. I sure did! The flavor, aroma and taste is just heavenly and I believe you gonna try it out in any of your festive celebrations, picnics or outings. This recipe is possibly among the best known and great keto burgers ever enriched by caramelized onions and brie.

Ingredients:

Mushrooms: - Butter (Two tablespoon)
             Sliced mushroom
             Salt

Burgers: Ground beef (two ibs)
              Salt (half teaspoon)
              Ground   pepper   (half
teaspoon)
              Brie cheese (4 ounce)

Onions: Salt (Half teaspoon)
              Olive oil (Two tablespoon)
              Sliced onions (one)

Preparation:

1. Caramelize your onions by heating it in a low heat medium container with olive oil, and then add your salt.

2. Heat gently for 30 minutes or until a soft and caramel brown color is observed. Don't allow it to become burnt or crisp.

3. Mix the pepper, salt and beef for your burger using your hand after which divide it into six equal portions.

4. Form nice patties with each portion half and on each of the patty top, put some of the onions and brie.

5. Cook your burger for 8 minutes on the pre-heated grill till it attains a temperature of 130 degrees Fahrenheit on the thermometer. Then, bring it down from heat and allow for 7 minutes to cool.

6. Cook the mushroom till it becomes brown and tender on both sides and then put it onto the cooked burgers.

7. Serve and enjoy your meal.

I.   YOGURT SAUCE WITH CHICKEN SOUVLAKI

OVERVIEW:

This meal which is a low carb, paleo, keto and Alkins diet friendly with a lot of flavors enriched with fresh oregano, garlic and lemon which can be easily seared or baked. This low carb recipe can be prepared easily and is equally ideal to arrange for any celebration or outing. The sauce highly complements the chicken though the chicken is good to go on its own if you aren't strong enough preparing the yogurt sauce.

Don't know how you guys feel about it buh to me, this diet is very simple and cooks fast giving you much time for other things on your schedule and time to even hang out with your loved ones outdoors.

Ingredients:

For your yogurt sauce, you need the following:

1. Lemon juice (one teaspoon)
2. Minced garlic (one teaspoon)
3. Fresh oregano (one teaspoon)
4. Greek yogurt (Three-quarter cup)
5. Granulated sugar (half teaspoon)

For the Chicken, you need the following:

1. Chicken breast (One Kilogram)
2. Olive oil (three tablespoon)
3. Lemon juice (Three tablespoon)
4. Red wine (One tablespoon)
5. Minced garlic (Four cloves)
6. Kosher salt (Two tablespoon)

7. Black   pepper   (one-quarter
   teaspoon)
8. Dried thyme (Half teaspoon)

Preparation of Yogurt Sauce

1. Mix every ingredients of your yogurt sauce very well.
2. Stir till you get your preferred seasoning and then serve with your chicken souvlaki.

Preparation of Chicken Souvlaki

1. Mix your lemon juice, red wine, olive oil, garlic, salt, oregano, pepper and dried thyme together in a dish.

2. Mix very well after adding the chicken strips into your marinade; then refrigerate for 60 minutes.

3. Grill your chicken after pre-heating for 5 minutes.

4. Enjoy your meal with the yogurt sauce.

J. SHRIMP OF PESTO

OVERVIEW:

This dish is awesome and perfectly good that can serve as repertoire in every festive occasion. This is indeed an easy delicacy that can make your Christmas or events wow!

INGREDIENTS:

1. Frozen and fresh shrimp (24 oz)
2. Pesto sauce (Half cup)

PREPARATION:

1. Bring about 8 skewers and soak in water for 45 minutes.
2. Use a foil and line the baking sheet; Toss your shrimp properly in a medium dish using your pesto sauce.(this is to coat it)
3. The pesto-coated shrimp should be threaded onto the skewers. (you can then spoon any sauce remaining on top of the shrimp).

4. The shrimp should be broiled for 5 minutes on either side till it becomes opaque.

5. Enjoy your meal

Each serving contain 38g protein, 0.6g fibre, 508mg sodium, 0.2g sugar, 3g carbohydrates and 36g fats.

K. THE RIBS JERK BARBEQUE

OVERVIEW:

I have every assurance that you will love this spicy, sweet and tender low carb diets enriched with amazing nutrients and good to be used for any festive events because they are duper super delicious

INGREDIENTS:

1. Pork ribs (one rack)
2. Caribbean jerk seasoning (half cup)

Sauce Ingredients:

Tamari (one quarter cup)

Soya sauce

Water (one-quarter)

Fresh ginger (Two tablespoon)

Orange zest (Two tablespoon)

Orange juice (One-quarter cup)

White vinegar (one quarter cup)

Worcestershire sauce (One)

Rice wine vinegar (two tablespoon)

Sugar substitute (Paleo/honey) (Three tablespoon)

Xanthan gum (one teaspoon)

PREPARATION:

1. Use the jerk seasoning to coat the ribs very well and bake for 120 minutes at 330 degrees Fahrenheit.

2. Mix the ginger, water, soy sauce, white vinegar, Worcestershire sauce, orange zest, rice wine vinegar and dizon mustard in a medium and boil for 10 minutes.

3. Remove the ginger and orange zest by straining your sauce, and then add the sweetener and xanthum gum. Then whisk.

4. The cooked ribs should be coated very well with the sauce for 45

minutes and heat at a temperature of 380 degree Fahrenheit.

5. Rest for 15 minutes, serve and enjoy.

This dish has six servings with each serving containing 20g fat, 3g carbs and 34g protein and 320 calories.

CHAPTER FOUR

LOW CARB APPETIZERS AND SNACKS

1. Low carb cheese roll ups and salami.
2. Jalapeno poppers
3. Low carb Mediterranean eggs recipe.
4. Low carb perfect guacamole
5. Barbeque shrimp wrapped with keto-bacon
6. Hot dog keto-recipe
7. Low carb pups and dogs recipes.

A. LOW CARB CHEESE ROLL UPS AND SALAMI

OVERVIEW:

For your delicious and quick appetizers for your party or picnic, Bother yourself no more! Just with the preparation of this diet will give your guest the exact tasty delicacy that they will request many more of this recipe. You can make any manner of combinations but my profound dish is addition of both red peppers and banana peppers. This combination has sweet aroma and flavors when well-prepared despite any addition.

INGREDIENTS:

1. Chopped banana peppers (seven and half teaspoon)
2. Chopped red pepper (seven and half teaspoon)
3. Cream cheese (one and half ounce)
4. Salami (fifteen slices)

PREPARATION:

1. Sprinkle one teaspoon of your cream cheese and red pepper on each of your sliced salami.
2. Sprinkle on each 5 slices a teaspoon of your banana pepper after which the salami slices are folded onto it to form a taco.

3. Hold it firm with your toothpick and then close.

4. Enjoy your meal.

There are a total of 5 servings and each of the serving contains 2.80g of protein, 4.50g fats, 50 calories, 0.62g carbs and 2.55g fibres.

B. JALAPENO POPPERS

OVERVIEW:

Personally, I liked this recipe the very first day I ate it at a friend's party and since then, that has been my nicest choice of smookie for my family especially in any outings or parties.

Though there are members of my family who don't like eating spicy foods. This made me to be using red bell peppers which they do enjoy. These diets are really enjoyable when served hot and are the best choice of food for every party.

INGREDIENTS:

1. Jalapeno peppers (Ten)
2. Slices of Bacon (Ten)
3. Mini smokies or sausages (Ten)
4. Cream cheese (one cup)
5. Grated Monterey jack (one cup)
6. Chili powder (one teaspoon)
7. Minced shallots (two)

PREPARATIONS:

1. Make a lengthwise cut of your jalapenos and remove the

membrane and seeds with a spoon (there will be a hallow formed)

2. Make a proper mixture of your minced shallots, chili powder, Monterey jack and cream cheese and fill this jalapeno hallows with the mixture.

3. The smokie should then be placed onto the cream cheese while the bacon (Half slice) should be wrapped around your Jalapeno. If your bacon is not tightly held; a toothpick can be used.

4. Place on the oven for 2 hours at a temperature of 225 degree Fahrenheit or till your bacon turns brown.

5. Serve and enjoy your delicious recipe.

C. LOW CARB MEDITERRANEAN EGGS RECIPE

DESCRIPTION:

One funny way of getting any idea on recipe to prepare is by storming my fridge, take a look of what's remaining there and then mixing up various ingredients. That was exactly how I gave birth to this devilish egg recipe which I'm sure you will enjoy just the way my family and I were entertained by this wonderful recipe. Anyway, while preparing it, I was a little skeptical about it- I was not optimistic enough whether the egg yolk will go well with the flavors and if the color will be brilliant. Alas! The opposite was the case as I had an excellent flavor and color.

INGREDIENTS:

1. Large eggs (one dozen)
2. Mayonnaise (Half cup)
3. Dizon mustard (one teaspoon)
4. Chopped capers (one tablespoon)
5. Kalamata olives (one tablespoon))
6. Chopped tomatoes (one teaspoon)
7. Olive oil (one tablespoon)
8. Minced basil (Two tablespoon))
9. Caper brine (one teaspoon)
10. Pepper and salt.

PREPARATIONS:

1. Boil eggs for 8 minutes in a sauce pan; Allow eggs to stay in the hot water after boiling for a period of twenty minutes. (switch off source of heat)

2. Remove eggs from hot water and slice all the eggs into two equal halves carefully.

3. Bring out their yolks and mash properly in a bowl using a fork.

4. Mix your mustard, mayonnaise, capers, sundried tomatoes, basil, olive oil and caper brine properly in your food processor.

5. Into the egg yolks, put the above mixture. Add your pepper and salt to get your desired taste.

6. Serve and enjoy.

Each serving contains 80 calories, 8g fats and 6g proteins.

D. LOW CARB PERFECT GUACAMOLE

OVERVIEW:

The best low carb guacamole! It's very easy to prepare using salt, Serrano chiles ripe avocados, lime and cilantro. Ensure to use ripe avocados. That's the perfect trick for a good guacamole. Ensure adequate precautionary measures are taken while handling chiles by washing your hands thoroughly before touching your eyes.

INGREDIENTS:

1. Avocados (Two)
2. Kosher salt (Half teaspoon)
3. Lemon juice (one tablespoon)
4. Chopped cilantro (Two Tablespoon)
5. Minced red onion (two tablespoon)
6. Minced Serrano chiles (Two)
7. Chopped ripe tomatoes (Two)
8. Black pepper

PREPARATION:

1. Dissect your Avocado into 2 equal halves and then scoop out the seed and the flesh using your spoon into a medium sized bowl.

2. Mash your avocado with the fork and then add your lime juice and salt. (The essence of the lime juice is to provide a balance to the alkalinity and prevent the avocado from changing into a brown color)

3. Put your black pepper, cilantro, chopped onion and chiles and then use a plastic wrap to cover the guacamole surface and refrigerate.

4. Serve while cool and enjoy your guacamole.

E. BARBEQUE SHRIMP WRAPPED WITH KETO BACON

OVERVIEW:

This recipe is fully loaded with amazing flavors which will provide good and enriching diets that will leave you begging for more of these delicious diets.

INGREDIENTS:

1. Bacon (Eight)
2. Shrimp (Sixteen)
3. Sauce (Two tablespoon)
4. Water (Half cup)
5. Chipotle powder (Half teaspoon)

6. Lime juice (Two teaspoon)

7. Granulated sugar (One teaspoon)

PREPARATION:

1. In a heat-proved pan, boil the bacon till it becomes pretty brownish or for 5 minutes.

2. Mix your sweetener, lime juice, powder, water and the sauce in a medium pan.

3. Mix your prepared sauce with the precooked bacon and heat gently for about 5 minutes.

4. Dissect the bacon into about sixteen pieces after removing it from the sauce.

5. Inside your sauce, put the shrimp and allow for one minute.

6. Wrap bacon to each piece of the shrimp after removal from the sauce and then skewer.

7. Grill the skewers for a minute on each side while ensuring it didn't stick onto the pan.

8. Serve while warm and enjoy.

You can put more lime wedges if you want it that way.

F. HOT DOG KETO RECIPE

OVERVIEW:

This seems like your routine hot dog recipe. However these diets are wonderful and rich. I have eaten many different recipes even those that was used to prepare pigs in blanket. This led me to use my Keto Buns dough and I can assure you that it was amazingly great! After preparation, the dough was soft and fluffy on the inside while the outside was crispy.

INGREDIENTS:

1. Keto Buns (Half recipe)
2. Sausages (six)
3. Egg yolk (one)
4. Sesame or sunflower seeds (Two tablespoon)
5. Coarse salt (Half teaspoon)
6. Optional – Dijon mustard.

PREPARATIONS:

1. Use your mixer (e.g. Kenwood) to prepare the hot dog dough and wrap in a foil.

2. Refrigerate the wrapped foil containing the dough for a period of 40 minutes after the dough should be divided into 5 parts of equal size.

3. For each of the 5 dough, roll it into size of 15 inches with your wet hands (Ensure your hands are properly wet intermittently). The oven should be preheated at about 350 degree Fahrenheit.

4. Use your baking mat to line your baking sheet. Brush your egg yolk on all the hot dogs and sprinkle

your salt and seed. Heat on the oven for 50 minutes or till it becomes golden brown.

5. After baking, put it into your serving plate and enjoy with BBQ sauce, Ketchup or Dijon mustard.

The hot dog keto recipe has 6 servings and each contain 9.6g fibers, 20g protein, 25g fats and 350 calories

G. LOW CARB PUPS AND DOGS RECIPES:

OVERVIEW:

This recipe is not just for carnivals and fairs but can be done at home as well.

The diet is dairy-free, gluten-free and very easy to prepare.

INGREDIENTS:

1. Honeyville Almond flour (one cup).
2. Coconut flour (Three tablespoon)
3. Corn meal (Three tablespoon)
4. Salt (one-quarter teaspoon)
5. Erythritol (one tablespoon)
6. Baking powder (one quarter teaspoon)
7. Xanthan gum (one-quarter teaspoon)
8. Eggs (Three)
9. Oil (Two teaspoon)
10. Coconut milk(one-third cup)
11. Coconut flour (one tablespoon)

PREPARATION:

1. Put the chopstick and corn dog inside one end of your hot dog.

2. Preheat your oil in the frying pan and whisk all the corn dog dry ingredients together in a bowl and set it aside.

3. Do same with the wet ingredients and thoroughly mix carefully.

4. Sprinkle the coconut flour on the body of the hot dogs after it has been dried by a paper towel. Ensure the whole body is thoroughly coated which will make the batter to stick effectively.

5. Bake the corn dog in the oil for three minutes. Turn it intermittently with a pair of tongs. (Allow it to change to a brownish color before turning over to the other side).

6. After baking, put the corn dogs in a plate to enable them drain properly and then continue baking the other remaining hot dogs.

7. If any batter is remaining, add a corn dog batter into the oil to cook. Remove when a brownish color is formed. I tag it "pups". My kids love this meal for real.

Each serving contains 150 calories, 15g fat, 6g carbohydrates, 2g fiber and 3g protein

CHAPTER FIVE

LOW CARB SIDE DISH AND SALAD RECIPES

1. Potato salad low carb recipe
2. Low carb keto corn bread
3. Low carb cauliflower salad and shrimp
4. Pine nuts and feta with grilled zucchini.
5. Flow carb cobb salad
6. Broccoli salad
7. Balsamic reduction with salad of tomato mozzarella.

8. Pecan vinaigrette (toasted and grilled asparagus)

9. Smith apple slaw.

A. POTATO SALAD LOW CARB RECIPE

OVERVIEW:

This is a wonderful side dish that is prepared from combination of eggs, mayonnaise, pickles, root vegetables and boiled potatoes. One wonders if this is actually a salad. It is usually served with fried carp during festivals such as New Year and Christmas celebration. However on different occasions, I resorted to using different ingredients such as turnips or cauliflower which offered me amazing taste and flavors.

INGREDIENTS:

Vegetable Spices:

1. Apple cider vinegar (one tablespoon)
2. Black peppercorns (one teaspoon)
3. Bay leaves (Two)
4. Salt (Half teaspoon)

Salad and Dressing Ingredients:

1. Turnip (one medium)
2. Cucumbers (six)
3. Large eggs (six)
4. Onion (one)
5. Celery stalk (sliced)(one)
6. Mayonnaise (Three-quarter cup)

7. Dijon mustard (1 teaspoon)

8. Chopped parsley (Two tablespoon)

9. Vinegar (Two tablespoon)

10. Celery seeds (one teaspoon)

11. Salt (half teaspoon)

12. Black pepper.

PREPARATIONS:

1. Cook the eggs properly for Ten minutes (Be careful in cooking them so that they won't crack). After the 10 minutes, remove from hot water and put them into pan containing enough cold water.

2. Peel your turnip, celeries and rutabaga very well. Dice them to about an inch piece. Put them into a pot containing water after which

your vinegar, bay leaves, salt and peppercorns should be added to it.

3. Boil for twenty minutes or till your rutabaga becomes tender. Then dispatch into a colander and allow to cool.

4. Cut the onions thinly with the pickles properly diced. Add them into the bowl containing the mixture. Put your vegetables.

5. Remove the egg shell after it has become chilled. Ensure that the egg white didn't stick on to the egg shell.

6. Cut them (egg) into tiny units and put them into the bowl containing the mixture and vegetable. Pour

your vinegar and stir till it becomes well mixed and uniform. Put your Dijon mustard, mayonnaise, herbs, celery stalks and seeds and mix properly. Add your pepper and salt to bring out the unique taste.

7. Refrigerate for 24 hours. Serve and enjoy.

B. LOW CARB KETO CORN BREAD

OVERVIEW:

This is entirely a new recipe which you can prepare the way you like. The simple truth about this recipe is that it is very easy to prepare (within 10 minutes) and the ingredients are easily accessible. The nutrition contents are amazing with a lot of flavors and yummy tastes.

INGREDIENTS:

Dry Ingredients:

Bacon grease (one tablespoon)

Pork rinds (one-third cup)

Parmesan cheese (Three tablespoon)

Whey protein (Two tablespoon)

Baking powder (Half teaspoon)

Kosher salt (one pinch)

Wet Ingredients:

1. Sour cream (Two tablespoon)
2. Egg (one)
3. Extract of Amoretti popcorn (one-eight teaspoon)

4. Apple cider vinegar (one teaspoon)

PREPARATION:

1. Pour the bacon grease into the cornbread skillet which is heated for five minutes on oven at 400 degree Fahrenheit.

2. In a different dish, mix all the ingredients properly and do same to the wet ingredients.

3. Then, mix both the dry and wet ingredients together using your spatula till you get a smooth batter.

4. Bake gently on the oven for fifteen minutes at a temperature of 400 degree Fahrenheit.

5. Serve while warm with a lot of butter

6. Enjoy!

Each serving of this recipe contains 15g protein, 18g fats, 210 calories, 3g carbohydrates, 2g carbs and 0g fibers.

C. LOW CARB CAULIFLOWER SALAD AND SHRIMP

OVERVIEW:

Wow! It's another diet containing cauliflower. Right! You are surprised huh! I just can't imagine preparing a recipe without addition of this cauliflower. It's kinda an addiction though I do it basically because I'm aware about the amazing properties they contain (both as an immune system charger and anti-oxidant properties) including other features. So here we gonna see the ingredients for preparing this great recipe.

INGREDIENTS:

1. Cauliflower (one head)
2. Raw shrimp (one)
3. Olive oil (one tablespoon)
4. Cucumbers (Two)
5. Fresh dill (three tablespoon)
6. Olive oil (one-quarter)
7. Lemon Juice (one-quarter cup)
8. Lemon zest (two tablespoon)
9. Pepper and salt.

PREPARATION:

1. Peel the shrimps and cast onto a sheet. Fry using the olive oil and sprinkle with the pepper and salt. Fry for 8 minutes at a temperature 350 degrees till they become opaque.

2. Dissect your cauliflower into tiny pieces and heat in the microwave for five minutes. Ensure that they are cooked evenly. Allow to cool.

3. Cut the cucumbers into tiny pieces while the cauliflower and shrimp are cooling; after which the shrimp are dissected lengthwise.

4. Mix your cucumber, cauliflower and shrimp properly in a bowl and

put the chopped dill and lemon zest.

5. Add your lemon juice with the olive oil and stir to coat properly.

6. Put your pepper and salt seasoning.

7. Serve and enjoy your meal.

Each serving contains 220 calories, 13g fats, 5g carbohydrates and 18g protein.

D. PINE NUTS AND FETA WITH GRILLED ZUCCHINI

OVERVIEW:

This is another well-nourished diet that can be used to supplement your dinner. With a recipe of grilled zucchini, my celebrations are always awesome and mind-blowing.

INGREDIENTS:

1. Zucchini (Four pieces)
3. Olive oil (one tablespoon)
4. Oregano (one and half tablespoon)
5. Black pepper
6. Kosher salt
7. Lemon zest
8. Goat cheese (Three ounces)
9. Pine nuts (one quarter cup)
10.   Parsley leaves (one-quarter cup)

PREPARATIONS:

1. Pre-heat your grill and cut the zucchini in a lengthwise strip.

2. In a bowl, the zucchini should be mixed and coated by the olive oil. Then add your kosher salt, oregano and black pepper on either sides and allow for ten minutes.

3. Grill for 5 minutes on both sides and drizzle with more of the lemon juice and olive oil.

4. To the softened zucchini, add your pine nuts, goat cheese, parsley leaves and lemon zest.

5. Serve while warm and enjoy.

E. SESAME GINGER WITH NOODLES OF BROCCOLI STEM

OVERVIEW:

I am really intrigued by this recipe. Nowadays, noodles can be prepared by every family because of the ease of preparation. I was happy when I learnt that I can prepare noodles from broccoli stem. Many of the recipes I have observed usually employ broccoli noodles. Its stem is indeed ideal for combination with Asian flavors including ginger and I bet you, they are really enjoyable when served crunchy and fresh.

Note that you can employ a carrot peeler to cut the broccoli stems when the spiralizer is not available. Ok let's check up the ingredients and preparation.

INGREDIENTS:

1. Broccoli stems (4)
2. Sesame oil (Two tablespoon)
3. Soy sauce (one tablespoon)
4. Minced garlic (two cloves)
5. Grated ginger (one teaspoon)
6. Salt (half teaspoon)
7. Flakes of red pepper (one-quarter)
8. Sesame seeds (two tablespoon)

PREPARATION:

1. Use your spiralizer to form noodles from the broccoli stems

after washing thoroughly (carrot peeler can be used alternatively)

2. Put your noodles into a bowl and in another dish, mix your sesame oil, apple cider vinegar, soy sauce, salt, ginger, flakes of red pepper and pepper.

3. Pour the above mixture with the sesame seed onto the broccoli noodles and stir till you get a perfect combination.

4. Serve and enjoy!

This recipe has four servings and each serving contain 10.2g fats, 10.04g fibers, 4.05g protein and 7.62g carbs.

F. FLOW CARB COBB SALAD

OVERVIEW:

For every low carber, this gonna be a great recipe and meal for us. This healthy salad contains delicious egg toppings, onion, romaine lettuce, chicken, tomatoes, avocado, blue cheese and bacon. This meal is gluten-free and very ideal for every low carb dieter.

INGREDIENTS:

1. Arugula (Two and half ounces)
2. Egg (one)
3. Grilled chicken (Two ounces)
4. Bacon (Two and half)
5. Green onion (Half ounce)
6. Red pepper (One ounce)
7. Ripe avocado (one and half ounces)

8. Garlic (Three tablespoons)

PREPARATION:

1. Boil the egg gently for five minutes after which you allow to cool in cold water. (This is to ease the removal of the shell)

2. Cook your bacon till it becomes tender and crisp after which you add your romaine lettuce that has been properly chopped and stir to coat well.

3. Slice your red pepper, green onion, avocado, egg and the blue cheese crumbled.

4. In your desired perfect order or in strips, arrange your ingredients on the serving plate and enjoy.

This recipe has one serving and it contains 570 calories, 48g fats, 9g carbohydrates, 5g fiber and 35g protein.

G. BROCCOLI SALAD

OVERVIEW:

This diet is a great hit and it is very savory which makes it ideal and good for every low carb dieter. This recipe is best served after refrigerating for an hour which enables the flavor to combine properly against our earlier belief of serving it immediately.

INGREDIENTS:

1. Broccoli (six cups)
2. Chopped onions (one-quarter)

3. Mayonnaise (a cup)

4. Chopped almonds (Half cup)

5. Red vinegar (Two tablespoon)

6. Bacon (Eight slices)

7. Pepper and salt.

PREPARATION:

1. Mix your bacon, broccoli, almonds and onion in a medium dish.

2. In another different bowl, combine your vinegar, mayonnaise, pepper and salt very well.

3. On the broccoli mixture, sprinkle the dressing on it and mix very well till you get a homogenous coat.

4. Refrigerate for 60 minutes at least. Serve and enjoy.

H. BALSAMIC REDUCTION WITH SALAD OF TOMATO MOZZARELLA

OVERVIEW:

This is one of the quickest and easiest salads that can be prepared with a lot of ingredients that are available in stores such as tomatoes, mozzarella and basil and then dressed with this my favorite balsamic reduction. I'm definitely in love with this appetizer recipe.

INGREDIENTS:

1. Sliced tomatoes (Five)
2. Fresh sliced mozzarella cheese (Sixteen ounce)
3. Basil leaves
4. Olive oil

5. Black pepper and sea salt.

6. Balsamic vinegar (two cups) for balsamic reduction.

PREPARATION:

1. In alternate patterns, arrange in a vertical order the basil, mozzarella and tomato slices. Create about two rows.

2. Sprinkle your olive oil onto the salad after which you sprinkle your balsamic reduction as well.

3. Add your black pepper and sea salt and serve fresh.

For your balsamic reduction; cook your balsamic vinegar for half an hour or till the vinegar becomes like a thicker glaze.

4. Allow to cool and serve with your salad.

I. PECAN VINAIGRETTE (TOASTED) AND GRILLED ASPARAGUS

OVERVIEW:

This low carp recipe is very easy and quick to prepare and is my favorite dish. Though my pee (urine) has a funny smell after consumption of asparagus, I care less. Lol! I really enjoy the recipe most especially during summer.

INGREDIENTS:

1. Trimmed asparagus stalks (one)
2. Olive oil (One teaspoon)

   3. Kosher salt.

Vinaigrette Ingredients:

   1. Sriracha sauce (one teaspoon)

   2. Soy sauce (Two teaspoon)

   3. Wine vinegar.

   4. Granulated sugar (one sugar)

   5. Lime juice (one juice)

   6. Toasted pecans (two tablespoon)

   7. Grapeseed, avocado or olive oil (one-quarter cup).

   PREPARATION:

   1. Grill the asparagus on each side for few minutes after coating it with salt and oil.

   2. In a medium dish, mix the ingredients (for the vinaigrette)

apart from the pecans. Stir till it becomes properly combined. Put your nuts.

3. Add this prepared vinaigrette on this asparagus and enjoy your meal.

This recipe serving contain 18g fat, 170 calories, 4.03g carbs and 5g protein.

J. SMITH APPLE SLAW

OVERVIEW:

I love this low carb recipe because it's pretty easy and cheap (about 50 cent) to prepare, really has wonderful flavors with the refreshing aroma from the mint. The meal is amazingly gorgeous just a look at it will make you to start salivating. It's super healthy for everyone who desires a low-carb diet owing to the nutritious and weight reduction components present.

Ok let's look at the ingredients.

1. Lemon juice (one tablespoon)
2. Red cabbage (eight cups)
3. Chopped mint (one-quarter cup)
4. Avocado oil (one-quarter cup)
5. Vinegar (apple cider) (two tablespoon)
6. Granulated sugar/substitute (one tablespoon)
7. Chopped smith apples (Two cups)

PREPARATION:

1. Dissect the apples and mix with your lemon juice. In a bowl, mix your mint, cabbage and apple while in another separate dish; mix the sweetener, vinegar and oil together.

2. On this slaw, add the dressing. Mix to coat very well.

3. Refrigerate for two hours and serve while fresh.

Note: you can store it for about five days in the fridge but it is most enjoyable when eaten after 1 hour refrigeration. This recipe contains 7g fats, 85 calories, 6g carbs and 2g protein.

CHAPTER SIX

LOW CARB SAUCE, DRESSINGS AND CONDIMENT RECIPES.

1. Chocolate Barbeque sauce.
2. Mango Barbeque sauce with smoky tomato.
3. Vinaigrette herb with garlic.
4. Pesto of green radish
5. Barbeque sugar-free sauce.
6. Recipe of pesto
7. Gorgonzola butter with ribeye steak
8. 30 seconds Caesar dressing

A. CHOCOLATE BARBEQUE SAUCE

OVERVIEW:

This recipe is delicious and simple to prepare. Though there are many ingredients that are needed you just have to mix, boil and chill to get your sauce well-prepared. There are amazing flavors and aroma this recipe provides.

INGREDIENTS:

1. Ketchup (one cup)
2. Crushed garlic (two cloves)
3. Coconut oil (Two tablespoon)
4. Paprika (Two teaspoon)
5. Chili powder (one teaspoon)

6. Cocoa powder (Two tablespoon)

7. Apple cider vinegar (Two tablespoon)

8. Coconut aminos (Two tablespoon)

9. Erythritol (Two tablespoon)

10. Stevia extract (10 drops)

11. Black pepper and salt.

PREPARATION:

1. Cut your garlic after measuring the ingredients and transfer them into your saucepan.

2. Place the ingredients (butter ketchup, garlic, vinegar, coconut amino, cocoa powder, smoked salt, chili powder, smoked salt, chili powder, stevia, pepper and

erythritol) into a saucepan and mix properly.

3. Cook using low heat for ten minutes after which switch off the heat source.

4. You can then put it into the glass jar and refrigerate as long as you desire.

5. Serve and enjoy your meal.

B. SAUCE OF MANGO BARBEQUE AND TOMATO MIXTURE

OVERVIEW:

This is the best Barbeque sauce that is sugar free. Few weeks ago, I prepared it for my family and it was quite awesome.

It didn't caramelize but the ribs I made with the sauce were really tasty. This recipe was prepared first this Christmas. I shared it among my guests and friends and they couldn't guess there was absence of sugar if I didn't inform them.

INGREDIENTS:

1. Tomato puree (Two cups)
2. White vinegar (Half cup)
3. Dijon mustard (one-quarter cup)
4. Ketchup (one-quarter cup)
5. Sugar substitute (one-quarter cup)
6. Liquid smoke (one tablespoon)
7. Apple cider vinegar (one tablespoon)
8. Fish sauce (one teaspoon)

9. Lemon juice (two tablespoon)

10. Dehydrated onions (two tablespoon)

11. Ground coriander (one tablespoon)

12. Celery salt (half teaspoon)

13. Cayenne pepper (one teaspoon)

14. Smoked paprika (one teaspoon)

15. Garlic powder (one tablespoon)

16. Cinnamon (half teaspoon)

17. Allspice (half teaspoon)

18. Cardamom powder (half teaspoon)

19. Ground ginger (one teaspoon)

20. Ground cloves (half teaspoon)

21. Optional- Mango syrup (one tablespoon)

PREPARATION:

1. In your sauce pan, mix the whole ingredients above properly and steam for half an hour (till you achieve your desired texture)

2. Add your salt, taste till you get your desired preference.

3. Serve with your main dish and enjoy.

C. VINAIGRETTE HERB WITH GARLIC

OVERVIEW:

This meal is an ideal salad dressing and taste good with a lot of vegetables or mixed green and it poses a great flavor. You can decide to prepare this salad the old school way using your hand to emulsify it. Alternatively, use your food processor or a blender.

INGREDIENTS:

1. Olive oil (half cup)
2. Champagne vinegar (one-quarter cup)
3. Powdered erythritol (one teaspoon)
4. Lemon zest (one teaspoon)
5. Water (two tablespoon)
6. Salt.

PREPARATION:

1. When using your blender, first measure your ingredients into a dish and mix very well (i.e. the ingredients) till it emulsifies.
2. Serve and enjoy.

D. PESTO OF GREEN RADISH

INGREDIENTS:

1. Radish green (three cups)
2. Garlic (two cloves)
3. Pine nuts (one- quarter cup)
4. Parmesan cheese (one cup)
5. Olive oil (one-quarter cup)
6. Pepper and Kosher salt.

PREPARATION:

1. Mix the whole ingredients in your food processor container and blend properly to get a uniform mixture.

2. Add your pepper and salt. Then refrigerate.

E. BARBEQUE SUGAR-FREE SAUCE

OVERVIEW:

With this sauce carefully prepared, there is no need to check the stores for sugarless sauce because you can now prepare your own barbeque sauce. The meal is a real deal, easy to prepare and very tasty.

INGREDIENTS:

1. Tomato sauce (Fifteen Oz)

2. Onion powder (one tablespoon)

3. Tomato paste (Six Oz)

4. Salt (one tablespoon

5. Garlic powder (one tablespoon)

6. Yellow mustard (One and half tablespoon)

7. Erythritol (two tablespoon)

8. Vinegar (one quarter cup)

9. Molasses (one tablespoon)

10. Liquid smoke (one teaspoon)

PREPARATION:

1. Mix the whole ingredients in your bowl very well and heat gently till the sauce starts bubbling for fifteen minutes.

2. Serve immediately or dispense into a container and refrigerate for future usage.

The molasses and liquid smoke are optional but I do add them because of the flavor they contribute to the sauce.

F. RECIPE OF PESTO

OVERVIEW:

Making this sauce at home is not a herculean task but very easy. The dish is very better in every respect than those you buy in your stores. If you are worried about preparing fresh pesto for your family, then this should be a MUST-DO for you. All that is required is just your food processor and quite some ingredients and you're good to go.

INGREDIENTS:

1. Washed basil leaves (one cup)
2. Romano cheese or grated parmesan (one-quarter)
3. Olive oil (one-quarter cup)
4. Pine nuts (one-quarter)
5. Chopped garlic (three cloves)
6. Kosher salt (one-quarter teaspoon)
7. Black pepper (one-quarter teaspoon)

PREPARATION:

1. In the bowl of your food processor, mix all your ingredients till it combines very well

2. Store in the refrigerator and use whenever you desire.

G. GORGONZOLA BUTTER WITH RIBEYE STEAK

OVERVIEW:

If you are a lover of beef, then this sauce is right for you and your family or guests.

INGREDIENTS:

1. Ribeye steaks

2. Softened butter (Half cup)

3. Gorgonzola cheese (Two oz)

4. Parsley , chopped (one-quarter cup)

5. Crushed garlic (one clove)

6. Pepper and salt.

PREPARATION:

1. Heat gently your ribeye steaks with pepper and salt on each side.

2. On your seasoned steaks, pour your gorgonzola butter (chilled one) and allow for five minutes and serve.

To prepare your Gorgonzola butter: Mix your gorgonzola, butter, garlic and parsley in the food processor and then chill.

H. 30 SECONDS CEASAR DRESSING

OVERVIEW:

This rich creamy salad dressing is a perfect deal for your festivities. Within 30 seconds, you will have a full jar of this amazing dressing at your disposal. The meal is really spectacular and simple to prepare.

INGREDIENTS:

1. Pasteurized egg (one)
2. Olive oil (one cup)
3. Parmingiano Reggiano cheese (one-quarter cup)
4. Smashed garlic (one clove)
5. Lemon juice (four tablespoon)
6. Dijon mustard (one and half teaspoon)

7. Black pepper (half teaspoon)

8. Salt (half teaspoon)

9. Anchovy paste (one and half teaspoon).

PREPARATION:

1. Bring your oil and egg to room temperature; mix the whole ingredients in your mason jar

2. Insert your immersion blender inside this Mason jar and blend till all the whole dressings become emulsified. Taste and adjust your seasoning with salt, pepper, more lemon or anchovy as you desire.

3. Refrigerate and serve with your main dish.

NOTE: I use pasteurized eggs against the raw ones because the latter may contain bacteria which can cause issues and make you sick.

CHAPTER SEVEN

LOW CARB DRINKS

1. Low carb julep of chocolate mint.
2. Whiskey sour (low carb)
3. Float of root beer
4. Lime Rickey raspberry

A. LOW CARB JULEP OF CHOCOLATE MINT

OVERVIEW:

This low carb drink is amazingly good and will enable you to celebrate your Christmas and other events the southern style. You just need your fresh mint leaves which can be chocolate mint or any other regular mint you can get. This drink is light, refreshing and very classic to prepare on your picnics, derby day, Christmas, New Year or any other celebration. For the sweetener, I used a mixture of white stevia powder and erythritol which were very perfect. It was easier for me because chocolate mint was grown at my kitchen garden so I prefer using it than the traditional spear mint.

INGREDIENTS:

1. Mint leaves (chocolate) (Three)
2. Erythritol (one tablespoon)
3. Crushed ice
4. Kentucky Bourbon (one ounce)
5. Club soda (Two tablespoon)
6. Mint sprig (one).

PREPARATION:

1. In your tumbler, mash your erythritol and mint leaves using a spoon or mudder; put your crushed ice.

2. Put your club soda and bourbon on the ice and taste.

3. If you desire, put little stevia into it and your mint sprig.

4. Pour some erythritol on it and garnish.

5. Refrigerate and serve while cold.

B. WHISKEY SOUR (LOW CARB)

OVERVIEW:

Whiskey sour is one of the drinks I can't do without. Not that I drink a lot but I do take a cocktail sometimes to refresh myself. The ingredients needed are handy and easy to get from the stores.

INGREDIENTS:

1. Lime juice (one quarter cup)
2. Ice cubes (one cup)
3. Whiskey (Three Ounces)
4. Xylitol (two teaspoon)
5. Lime syrup (one teaspoon)

PREPARATION:

1. Mix the whole ingredients in your blender and mix gently till it becomes smooth.
2. Put it into a glass that is chilled and then use your lime slice to garnish.

C. FLOAT OF ROOT BEER

OVERVIEW:

This is a keto-friendly and low carb drink. It is very delicious especially taking it after your dinner or on a very sunny day. Oh my Gosh! It's so heavenly! The chillness will cool your body temperature and give you this relaxed mind. However, be very cautious while drinking because one can easily get drunk if care is not taken. So be careful!

INGREDIENTS:

1. Root beer (one cup)

2. Spiced rum (one ounce)

3. Whipping cream (two tablespoon)

4. Cube ice.

PREPARATION:

1. Mix all your ingredients into a container with your ice.

2. Shake very well to combine (about a minute).

3. Pour into your tumbler, refrigerate and enjoy.

This drink has about 170 calories, 0g fibers, 0g carbs, 0g protein and 10g of fat.

D. LIME RICKEY RASPBERRY

OVERVIEW:

Traditionally, lime rickey is composed with bourbon or gin with little sugar added. However, in the ones I prepared, I added raspberry syrup which is sugar-free and gives pleasant color and flavor. I also added a little mint leaves and lime. Indeed the drink is savory, enticing and mouth-watering.

INGREDIENTS:

1. Club soda (sixteen oz)
2. Raspberry syrup (four oz)
3. Limes (four)
4. Gin (six oz)

5. Mint leaves (eight)

6. Ice.

PREPARATION:

1. Mix your mint leaves and limes in about five glasses

2. Put your slub soda and your raspberry syrup (sugar-free)

3. Put the liquor you desire. I prefer gin but you can use vodka as well.

4. Mix very well and garnish with limes, raspberry and any mint leaf.

CHAPTER EIGHT

DESSERT RECIPES (LOW CARB)

1. Lemon bar dessert
2. Coconut fudge (white chocolate)
3. Cupcake floats of root beer.
4. Cake of strawberry mug
5. Cheesecake bar with peanut butter.

A. LEMON BAR DESSERT

OVERVIEW:

This is one of my desserts that I cannot do without. I use to gaze steadily at the coffee house or the bakery whenever I do pass those arenas with a quest to enter and have one. Sometimes, I do task my pocket to get one but I regret the next day after I become bloated from those sugar and gluten content. So I now decide that I will prepare my own keto-friendly, lemon bar that will be gluten and sugar-free. Alas! It was bomb. My friends ate and they are paying me to prepare it for them. Lol!

I'm pretty sure that you guys are going to be comfortable with this dessert.

INGREDIENTS:

Crust Ingredients:

1. Butter (six tablespoon)
2. Almond flour (two cups)
3. Sugar substitute (one-third cup)
4. Lemon zest (fresh) (one tablespoon)

Filling Ingredients:

1. Butter (half cup)
2. Sugar substitute (e.g. swerve) (half cup)
3. Lemon juice (half cup)

4. Lemon zest (one-quarter cup)

5. Yolks (six egg)

6. Xanthan gum (half teaspoon)

7. Gelatin (two tablespoon).

PREPARATION:

For Your Crust:

1. In your microwave, the butter should be melted: put your sweetener, almond flour, lemon zest and mix properly till it becomes well combined. Bake for a maximum of ten minutes at 350 degree Fahrenheit. Allow to cool.

For Your Filling:

1. In a pan, the butter should be melted on a low heat. Bring down from heat and add your lemon

zest, lemon juice and sweetener. Whisk till it becomes properly dissolved. Put your egg yolk and heat gently. Put the gelatin and xanthan gum till it becomes smooth and dissolved.

2. Sprinkle your filling on the crust and spread on it. Bake for fifteen minutes at a temperature of 350 degree Fahrenheit. Pour the swerve if you like and then serve.

B. COCONUT FUDGE (WHITE CHOCOLATE)

OVERVIEW:

This dessert is absolutely perfect. Preparing this dish is not quite easy as I failed many times before I got it right. It was a real challenge for me but finally, I became the master of the dessert. Hope you're curious to know how to prepare these irresistible bites.

INGREDIENTS:

1. Cacao butter (four ounces)
2. Coconut milk (one can)
3. Coconut oil (half cup)
4. Coconut butter (one cup)
5. Vanilla protein powder (half cup)
6. Vanilla extract (one teaspoon)
7. Coconut liquid stevia (one teaspoon)

8. Salt (pinch)

PREPARATIONS:

1. In your medium pan, the cacao butter should be melted under low heat.

2. Add your coconut oil, coconut milk and coconut butter and stir till it becomes absolutely smooth.

3. Bring down from heat source and put your stevia, vanilla extract, protein powder and salt.

4. On your parchment paper with dimension of 8 x 8, put this mixture into it and sprinkle with your coconut flakes as you wish.

5. Refrigerate for about five hours and enjoy.

C. CUPCAKES FLOATS OF ROOT BEER

OVERVIEW:

This is a gluten-free low carb cupflakes composed of chocolate and topped with a frosting of cream. Honestly, I had a fun time preparing these cupcakes. With my extract of root beer that has been crying for long in my refrigerator to be used, I had no other option than to apply use it for the preparation of this unique dessert.

Watch out and see how I prepared this amazing recipe.

INGREDIENTS:

1. Cacao powder (one-quarter cup)
2. Almond flour (two cups)
3. Whey protein (unflavored) (one-third cup)
4. Baking powder (two teaspoon)
5. Baking soda (half teaspoon)
6. Xanthan gum (half teaspoon)
7. Salt (one-quarter teaspoon)
8. Butter (five tablespoon)
9. Sweetener (one-third cup)
10. Eggs (two)
11. Extract of root beer (two teaspoon)

12. Stevia extract (one-quarter teaspoon)

Frost Ingredients:

1. Whipping cream (one cup)

2. Swerve sweetener (one-third cup)

3. Extract of vanilla (half teaspoon)

PREPARATION:

To Prepare your Cupcakes –

1. Use your paper liners and place them on the muffin pan which is on the oven pre-heated to 330 degree Fahrenheit.

2. In a small dish, mix your cocoa powder, almond flour, whey protein, baking soda, xanthan gum, and salt.

3. In a medium dish, put the erythritol and butter. Beat till it becomes creamy. Put the extract of root beer, eggs and extract of stevia.

4. Put your almond flour and mix very well and pour the well-mixed compositions into the muffin cups. Bake for thirty minutes and then allow cooling in your pan.

To prepare your frost:

1. Mix your vanilla extract, erythritol (powdered) and cream in a medium dish and beat to get a perfect mixture.

2. Spoon or pipe into your cupcakes.

This dessert has twelve servings and each has about 25g fats, 270 calories, 80g protein, 3g fiber and 4g carbs.

D. CAKE OF STRAWBERRY MUG

OVERVIEW:

This is an easy and delicious microwaveable recipe that is enriched with a lot of flavors and nutrition. It is just very ideal for every low carber.

INGREDIENTS:

For Your Cakes:

1. Butter (two tablespoon)
2. Sugar substitute (two tablespoon)
3. Almond flour (one-quarter cup)
4. Coconut flour (one tablespoon)

5. Egg (one)

6. Strawberries (one-quarter cup)

7. Baking powder (half teaspoon)

8. Vanilla extract (half teaspoon)

For Your Strawberry Cream:

1. Whipping cream (half cup)

2. Strawberries (two tablespoon)

3. Sugar substitute (one tablespoon.

PREPARATION:

For Your Cake:

1. First, the butter should be melted in your microwave saucepan; then put the other cake ingredients and mix properly.

2. Divide your batter into 2 coffee mugs and heat for two minutes.

Ensure you don't overcook or rather you can bake it for twenty minutes on the oven at a temperature of 380 degree Fahrenheit.

For Your Strawberry Cream Preparation:

1. Mix your whipping cream, sweetener and strawberry in a small bowl. Put the strawberry mixture together with the whipped cream.

2. Pipe or spoon it on top of your mug cakes.

3. Enjoy your meal.

E. BARS OF CHEESECAKE WITH PEANUT BUTTER:

OVERVIEW:

This is a great meal composed with cream cheese, vanilla, peanut butter, egg and a sweetener. Owing to the fact that I cherish peanut, preparing this recipe was of utmost interest to me because I was happy that at least, I will produce peanuts that contains low carb but rich in nutrition.

Let's look at the ingredients:

INGREDIENTS:

For Peanut Butter:

1. Cream cheese (one package)

2. Peanut butter (two servings)

3. Vanilla (one teaspoon)

4. Egg (one)

5. Sugar substitute (half cup)

Toppings:

1. Crushed peanuts (Twenty-eight grams)

2. Peanut butter (one tablespoon)

3. Coconut oil (one teaspoon)

4. Hershey's chocolate (one)

5. Coconut oil (one teaspoon).

PREPARATIONS:

1. Let the cream cheese be softened by your microwave first.

2. Mix all your whole ingredients in a bowl and bake for thirty

minutes at a temperature of 300 degree Fahrenheit.

3. Pour more chocolate and peanut butter on top with your crushed peanuts

4. Refrigerate for at least five hours and then, dissect them into bars.

INGREDIENTS:

For Your Chocolate Crust:

1. Almond flour (one cup)

2. Coconut flour (two tablespoon)

3. Xanthan gum (half teaspoon)

4. Salt (one-quarter teaspoon)

5. Bakers chocolate (two servings)

6. Butter (one-quarter cup)

PREPARATION:

1. The oven should first be pre-heated to a temperature of 350 degree Fahrenheit.

2. The sweetener should be added to the baker's chocolate (which is already melted and mixed very well. The sweetener too should be added into the molten butter and thoroughly mixed.

3. Mix your dry ingredients very well (coconut flour, almond flour, salt and xanthan gum).

4. Using a mixer, mix properly the butter with the chocolate and blend till the whole ingredients are properly mixed.

5. Put the mixture into an 8 x 8 pan and bake for ten minutes at a temperature of 350 degrees.

6. Refrigerate for thirty minutes and   then   cut.

CONCLUSION

Hello Dear reader, I believe that this book has helped you in your quest for a healthy belly using the amazing diets that are detailed here.

I still have other good resources that can help you or a friend.

Thanks for reading!

Made in the USA
San Bernardino, CA
02 June 2018